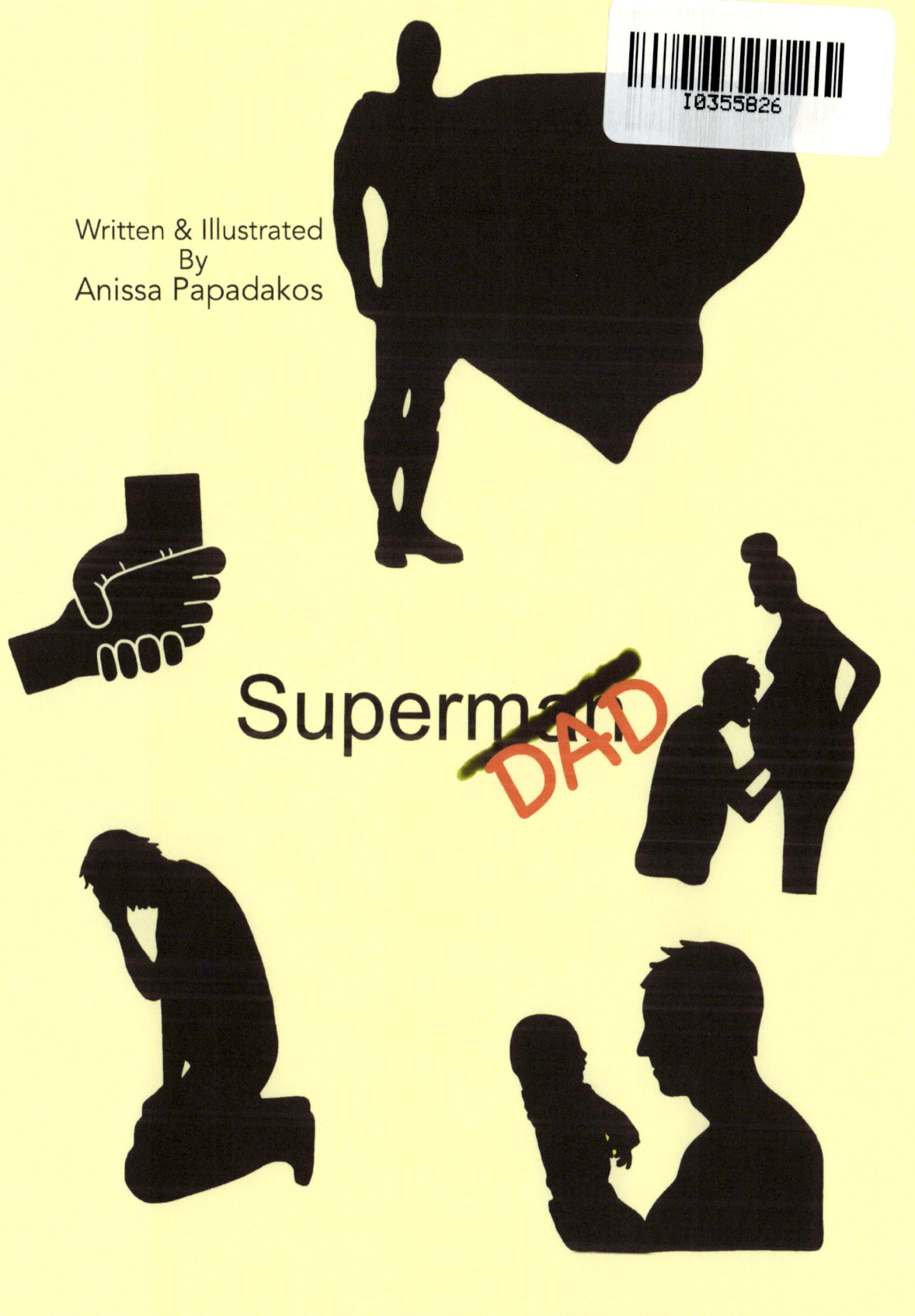

Written & Illustrated By
Anissa Papadakos

Super~~man~~ DAD

Copyright ©2021 Magic Walls & Canvas. All rights reserved.
ISBN: 978-0-6484235-3-9

All rights reserved. No part of this publication may be reproduced or transmitted in any form or by any means, electronic or mechanical, including photocopying, recording, storage in an information retrieval system, or otherwise, without the prior written permission of the publisher, unless specifically permitted under the Australian Copyright ACT 1968 as amended.

Written by Anissa Papadakos
Illustrated by Anissa Papadakos
Text Copyright © Anissa Papadakos
Illustration Copyright © Anissa Papadakos

Visit: www.magicwallsandcanvas.com
Facebook : Anissa Papadakos
Instagram : magic walls and canvas

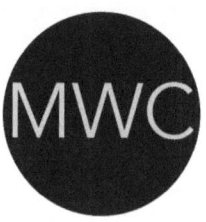

Anissa wishes to thank her wonderful editor, Kat Pagan, for her extraordinary work in transforming her manuscript into a poetic piece of art.
Facebook: Pagan Proofreading
Instagram: kat_m_pagan

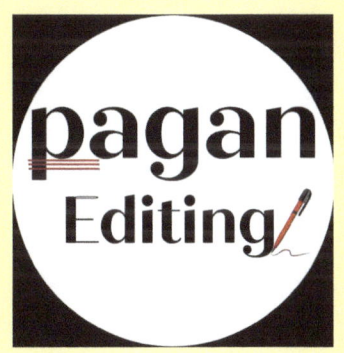

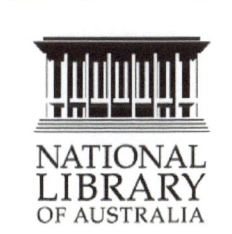

A catalogue record for this book is available from the National Library of Australia.

To all fathers out there
(young & old or soon to be)

You're all a Superman

Special Thanks to my Husband & Family

Other Books By Author:

The Adventures of Mr C
The Brochure Lied

Dear Dad aka Superman,

Who would have known fatherhood would be so difficult?

Who would have known?

When I became a father, the problems began almost immediately. And they began with me. I just didn't want to admit to the emotions that I was feeling. The anxiety and the fear.

"Why should I?" I thought at the time.

"I am a MAN."

"I am not supposed to show cracks in my armour."

Life changed forever the moment I saw my baby in the delivery room. To be honest, I felt strange. I didn't know how I was going to love this baby. My baby. I felt no love and no connection. And that scared me.

It was all different during the pregnancy. I didn't feel anxious and I didn't feel fear. Maybe it was due to being busy with work and life in general. I was constantly having fun, being active, and enjoying the world, my wife and my friends. Or maybe it was simply due to the baby not being here yet—an "out of sight, out of mind" type of thing.

When the midwife handed me my baby, to be honest, I felt sick to the stomach. I felt like this baby was not mine, and I also felt like this baby didn't want me. In the hospital ward, they encouraged skin to skin time to help you bond. For some reason or another, that did not help me and I didn't understand why.

Today, when I look back, I should have voiced what I felt in that moment. I should have said something but I didn't. I didn't because I was brought up believing that I should avoid showing my pain. Growing up we looked up to "Hard Men" who didn't show their emotions. And at that moment, I was feeling emotional and I was feeling weak. I kept telling myself I had to "Man Up" and everything would be okay. But it never was.

I thought going home was going to be better. In fact, life got worse and I slowly spiralled into depression. You see, our daughter did not sleep and she cried a lot. To make matters worse, my wife was not in a good place either... mentally. So, I had no choice but to hold the fort, and family, together.

I found, over time, my patience was beginning to dwindle. I didn't want to be around my wife and I certainly didn't want to be around my baby. I just didn't want to be home. I found myself staying late at work and going back in early. And because of this, I felt like a "bad dad".

I became bitter at life and at everyone.

Bitter at my family because they were too hard to deal with.

Bitter at my friends because no one called me.

Bitter at the fact that I didn't go out anymore.

Bitter that I stopped pursuing my interests and hobbies.

Bitter that everyone else had the perfect baby.

Bitter that everyone else felt love for their child or children.

Bitter that everyone else was happy when I was miserable.

I didn't think that I could tell my wife how I was feeling. And I didn't want to risk it impacting on her fragile mental health. So, I suffered in silence.

I suffered to the point that I had a complete breakdown in my car at work. I couldn't walk inside, let alone get out of the car. I just sat there in the driver's seat, shaking and crying, with suicidal thoughts running through my mind. After I calmed down, I knew something had to be done. I needed to get some help.

That night, my wife and I cried together and held each other for the first time in many months. I felt for the first time that she could see the tremendous effect this was having on me too. I felt validated by her simply recognising my pain. Slowly but surely, the dark cloud which had descended upon us began to lift. We started to heal by speaking up and by getting help from first our General Practitioner and then our counsellors.

I was totally unaware men/fathers could develop postnatal depression. To be honest, at the time, I didn't even know what it was. Through my journey, I just thought I was being strong for everyone, which in the end wore me out. But being strong means being aware of how you are functioning and asking for help when you are struggling.

Love From,

One Superdad to Another

Dear Amazing Hubby aka Superman,

How beautiful is parenthood even though it is filled with many bumps along the way? There are good days and there are bad days. Sometimes, the good days are tarnished by the bad days. And those days are hard. The good thing is we are not alone and we will get through this... together.

When we first found out we were expecting, it was complete illation. We were ecstatic. But something changed at that moment—it was life. The focus shifted to the baby in my belly. And for some reason, the spotlight on you, daddy, switched off while it only dimmed on me.

Now, I know that should not have happened. Your spotlight should have shined brightly too. As a wife and a mother, I now understand your mental health is just as important as mine—pre and postpartum. I now understand why you were so distant from us, and I don't blame you nor do I fault you.

It was hard to adjust to our new way of life when the baby arrived. You not only had to look after my well-being as well as your own, but you also had to look after and feed our baby. All this while paying bills and going to work after a hard and sleepless night. That is stressful.

Thank you for looking after us while you stressed about your job.

Thank you for looking after us while you felt doubt about your capacity as a father.

Thank you for being strong even though within, you were falling apart.

If only I or someone else would have known sooner, we could have helped you. We could have held you. We could have dusted off your cape and reminded you how fantastic you are.

You still would have been our superhero if you told us you were hurting.

You still would have been our superhero if you asked for help because you were struggling.

Each time you fell, you dusted off your cape and kept on moving forward for us—The Family.

Even at that moment when you showed the cracks in your armour and asked for help, you dusted off your cape and kept on moving forward for us—The Family.

It is common for dads to ignore their own mental health because they feel they need to be strong for their families. But being strong means being aware of how you are functioning and asking for help when you are struggling.

So, thank you, Superdad, for being strong and for dusting off your cape.

Love,

Wonder Woman

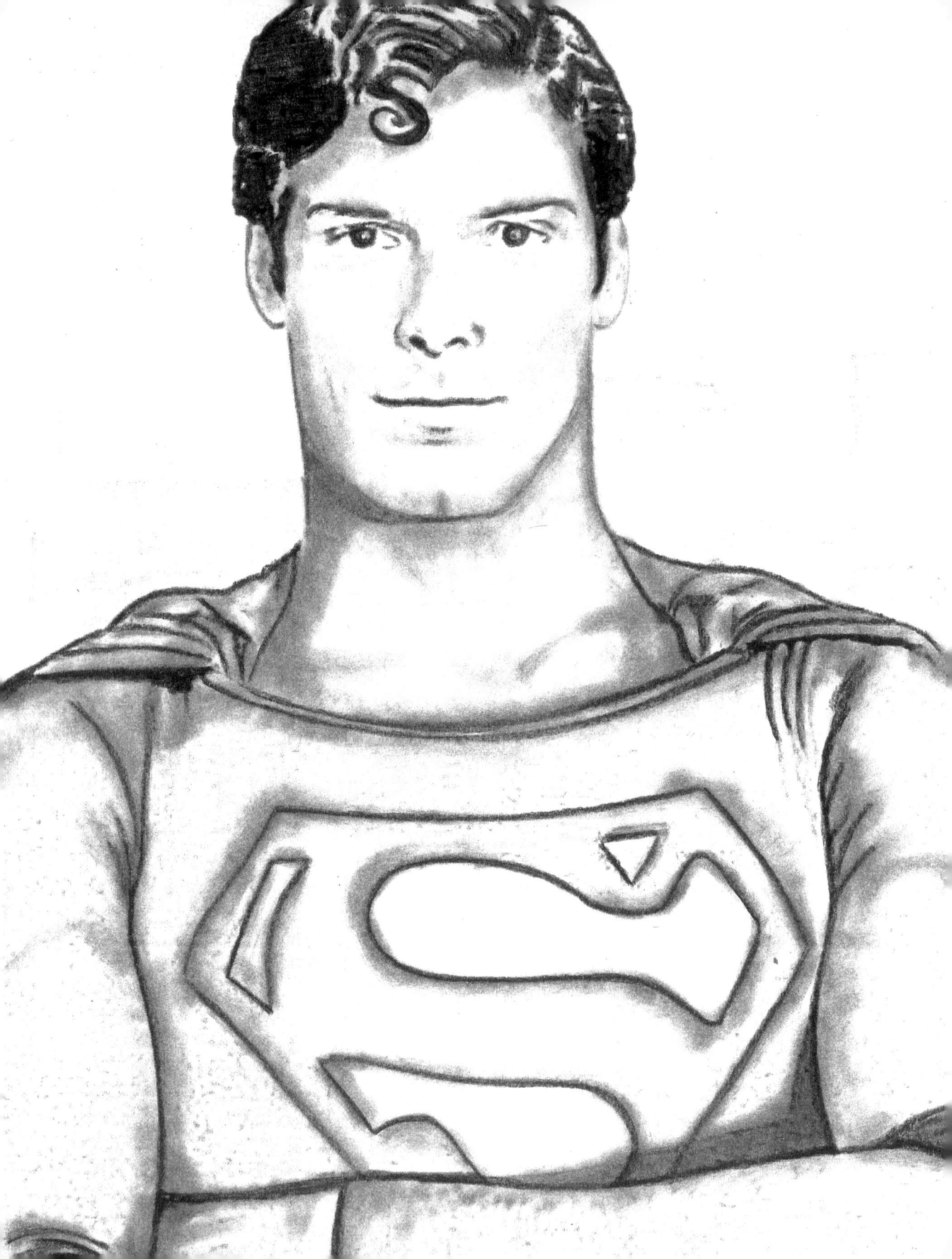

My name is Superman.
Hear me roar!
I am a good-hearted man who is fit right down to the core.
I keep myself as busy as a boy can be.
I am successful and even a great Hubby.

I am a lucky man; yes, I am.
Not because of my success,
Or by the Rolex on my hand.

You see, I am lucky as I married an absolute gem.
She is strong, a heroine.
She is my Wonder Woman.

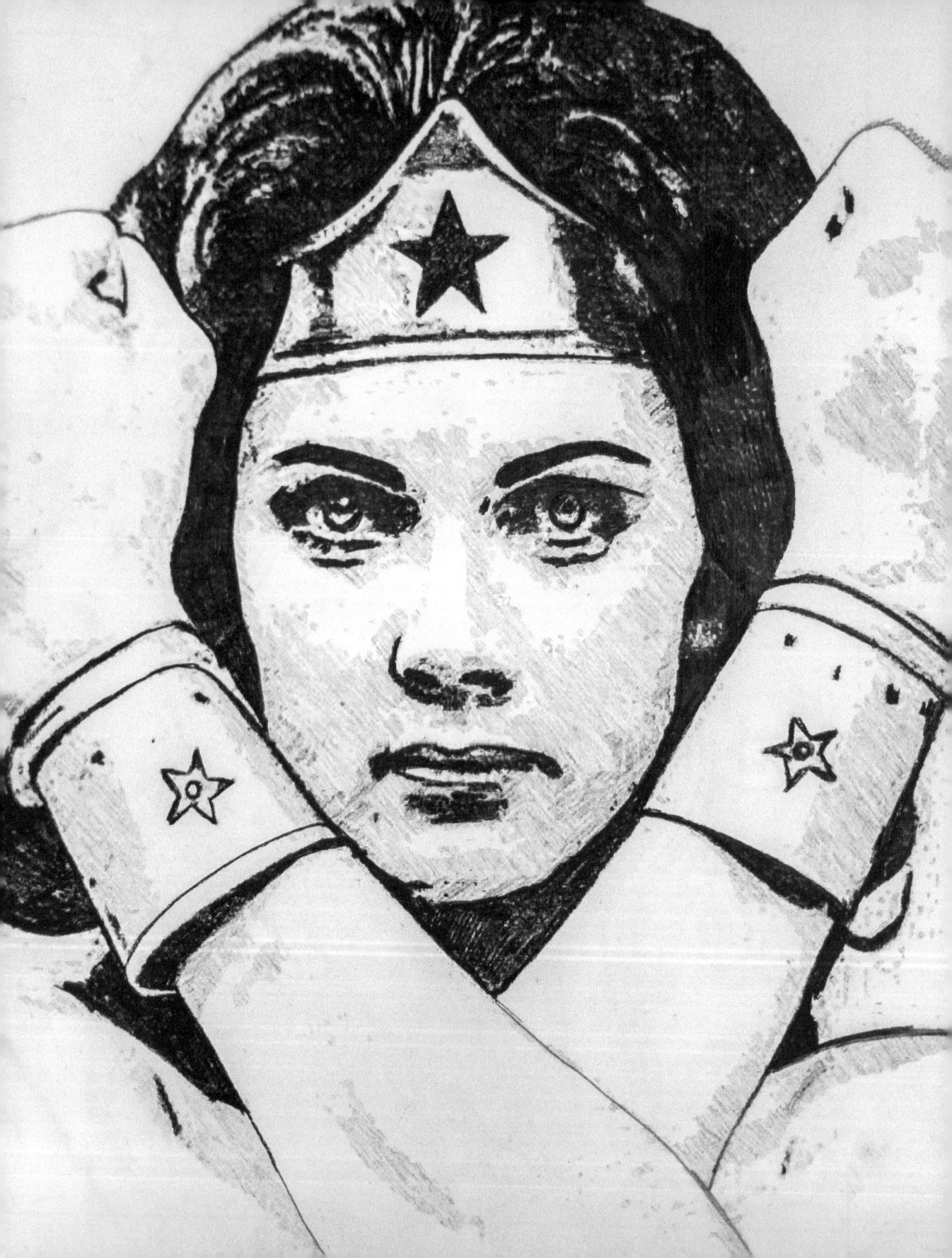

Wonder Woman is very beautiful,
As beautiful as a flower can be.
She is strong, certainly at times, stronger than me.

She helps me to be my best,
Always steering me back,
When I have veered right off the track.

She holds my hand when I am hurting.
She tends to my wounds when I feel defeat,
And always encourages me to stand tall on my own two feet.

I love life.
I love to have fun.
I love to be active and enjoy the sun.

I love to socialise with my friends,
By having a few drinks at the pub,
Or a BBQ on the weekends.

I am very sporty; yes, I am.
I love the footy with its rush and adrenaline.

The gym is a favourite place of mine,
Where I love to work out and pump my iron.
It gives me confidence about me,
And it's the place where I flex and look at my booty.

Last but not least,
I love to wine and dine my greatest love.
No, that's not my biceps…
But Wonder Woman, you schmuck!

We felt happy.
We felt great.
So far, we had everything that we wanted to date.

We even spent time travelling the world.
We visited exotic places from all four corners of the world.

But amongst all the sunshine and fun,
We felt our party of two was becoming a little bit dull.
So, one night as we cuddled together,
We decided to take the next step…
A step which surely, we wouldn't regret.
Because having a baby is so much fun,
That is what is said by everyone.

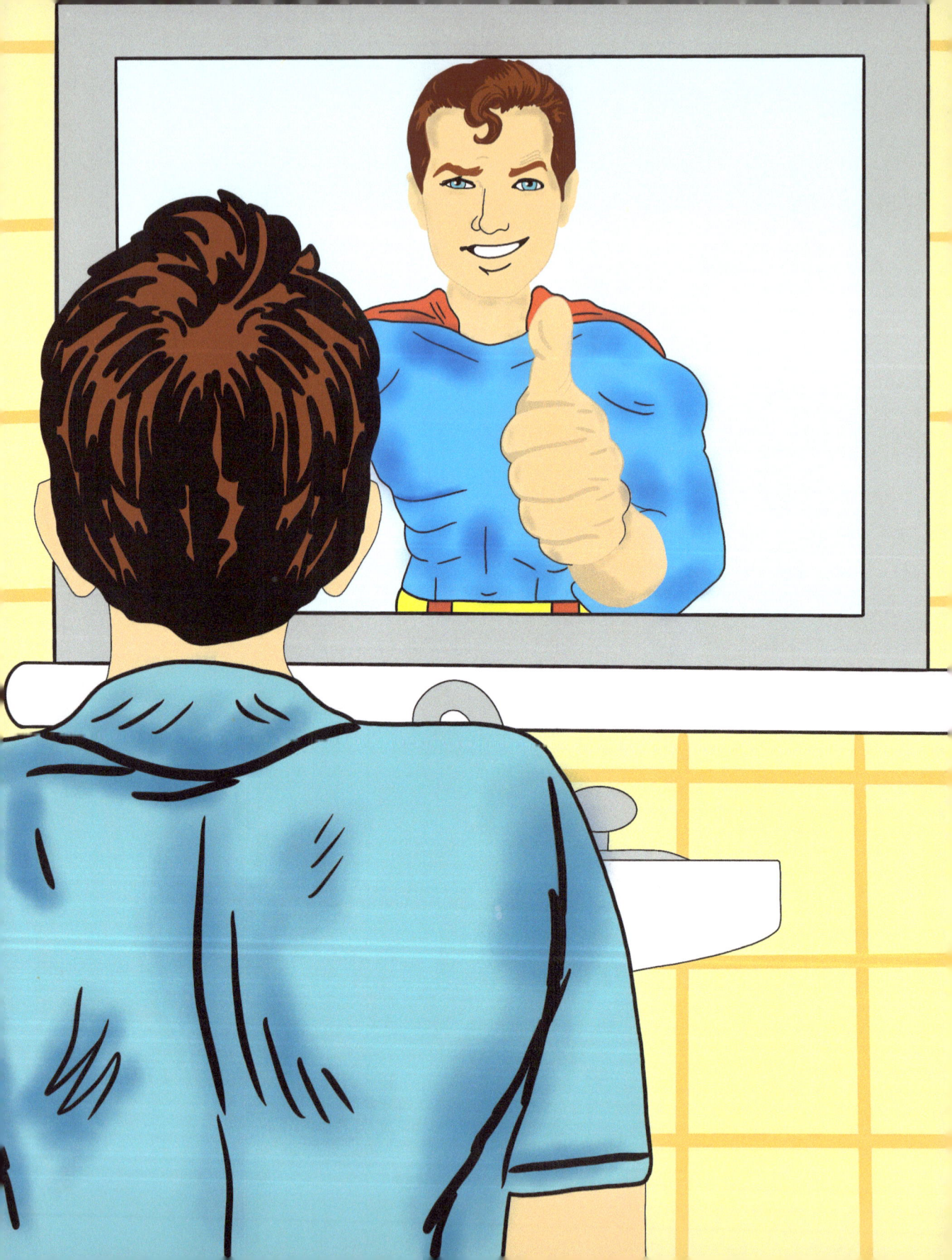

REASSURANCE

If only I could go back to that moment,
The moment we decided to take the next step,
I would tell myself that:

1. What I am feeling is normal and not abnormal
2. I am strong and confident
3. I am Superman

I would tell myself to go seek out people who could give me genuine advice,

People who could reassure me when I felt down and in doubt,

People who could remind me of how strong I am inside and out.

Then, on those bad days, I would be able to dust off my cape,
And look in the mirror and say: Superman, You Got This, Mate!

It didn't take long,
Not long at all,
To find that our party of two would soon be welcoming one more.

We were so happy.
We were so elated.
It was just incredible for us to believe that soon we would become parents.

You see, my beautiful Wonder Woman had already started to glow.
There was just something different about her from head to toe.
I couldn't quite pick it out.
It was difficult to see.
Perhaps it was her smile, which for some reason,
Looked upside down at times to me.

I didn't feel different…
Not me, no way!
I continued to work and even to play.

By play, I mean I socialised,
A beer with the boys or an evening at the footy every Friday night.

I even continued to exercise.
To remain fit and strong was important—oh my, that's no surprise!

But honestly, it was important for me…
As it allowed me to recharge my batteries.
It cleared my head of all negative thoughts.
It gave me the energy to take it all.
And take it all, I did.
I worked like a robot—sharp and quick!

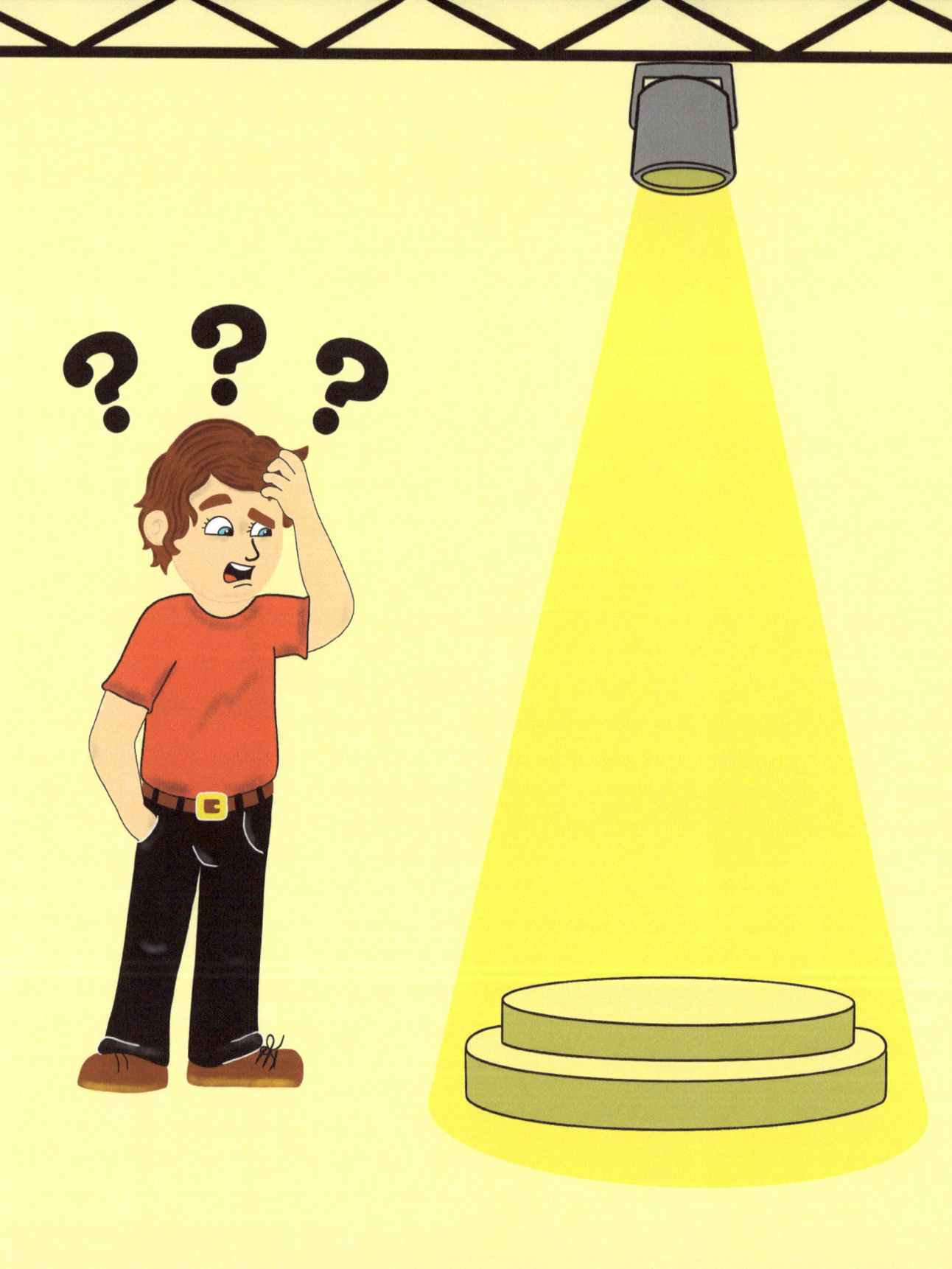

After all the day's work is done,
I liked nothing more than to be at home,
Resting with my loved ones.

I hadn't seen or chatted with you all day.
There are so many things I just wanted to say:
How are you feeling?
How is Bub?
Have you felt a kick or maybe a shove?

But as I sat there listening,
I realised that all this time not one question was directed to me.
Where is the spotlight?
Where can it be?
It certainly isn't shining down on me…
Doesn't anybody want to hear how all this affects me?

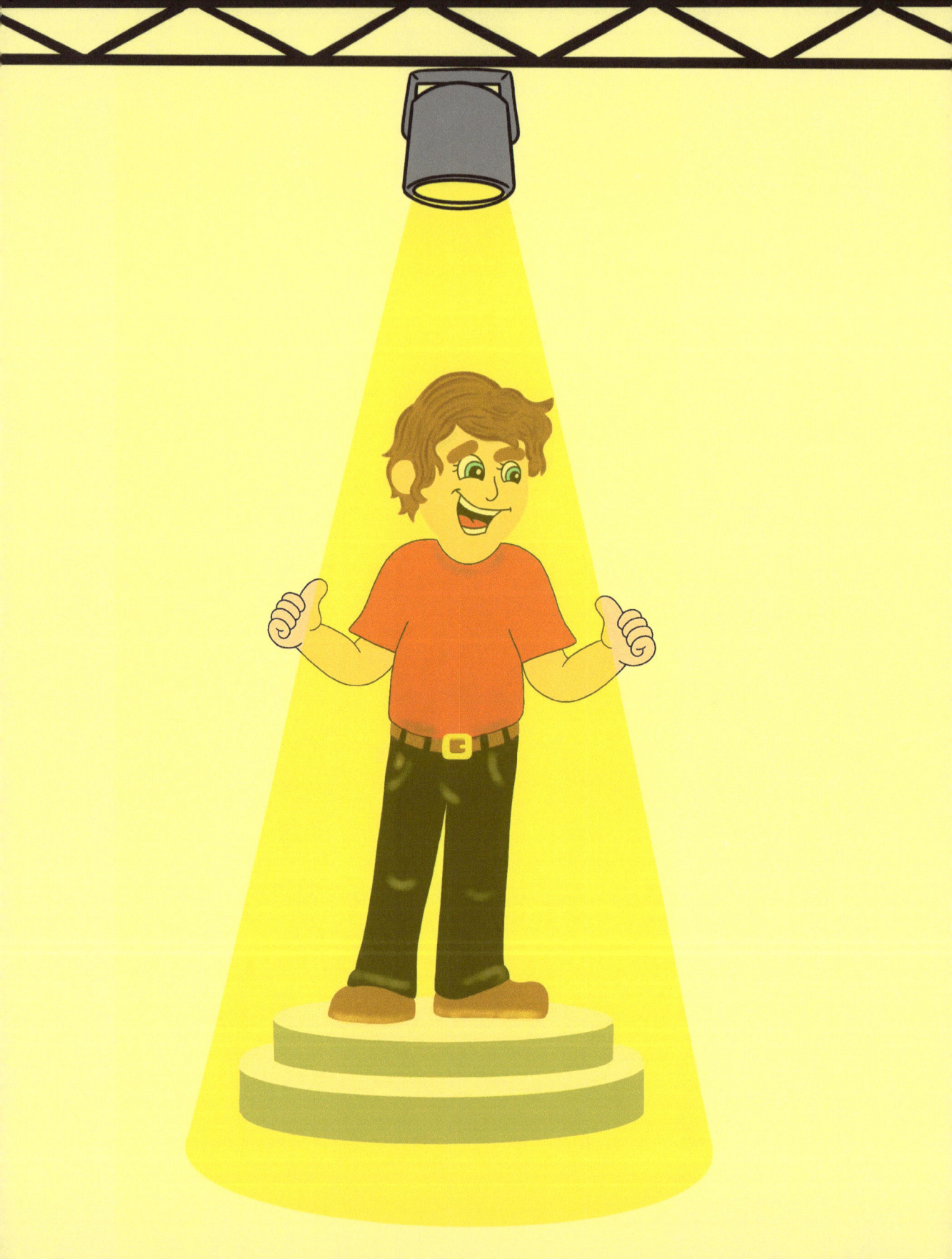

REASSURANCE

If only I could go back to that moment,
The moment when I started feeling like a mess,
I would tell myself that:

1. What I am feeling is normal and not abnormal
2. I am strong and confident
3. I am Superman

I would tell myself to go stand up and speak.
Speak up about how you feel.
Keeping it bottled up inside will never help you to heal.

Yes, you do matter, Superman.
You matter in every way.
The spotlight does also shine down on you, so please don't close up, mate.

Speak your heart's worries.
Shout them all out.
Your feelings do matter and they are not a weakness, no doubt.

So, if you feel the spotlight has shifted,
Shifted right away,
Make sure you grab it, Superman, and shine it your way.

The day you came into the world, my baby,
Was a day like no other.

Your mother and I were so excited when her water broke.
It meant you were not far away from your first cuddle and cheek stroke.

Wonder Woman pushed;
She pushed as hard as can be.
And with that last push,
You popped right out and started to scream at me.

In that moment, I did shed a tear,
A tear of pure joy.
Your screaming was not horrendous but music to my soul.

It was such a proud moment,
Very proud for me, as I gladly took the scissors, which were offered to me.
You see, it was my duty to cut you free.

And as I stood there cutting through what felt like tough chewie residue,
I just couldn't wait to cuddle you, my precious little booboo.

Then finally, after you were all bundled up,
They placed you in my arms…

And I felt cheated, just my luck.

Why did I feel this?
I did not know.
I loved you dearly just a second ago.

What possibly could have happened?
Where did my love for you go?
Am I simply dreaming up this horror show?

But as I stood there holding you,
I sincerely asked why don't I love you?
You didn't answer me as I knew you couldn't.
I was just surprised that my feeling of love had withered.

I am so confused; yes, I am.
Why didn't I get that overwhelming feeling of love, like every other dad can?
They all speak about it; yes, they do.
They just light right up in front of you.
Mmm, maybe what they say is not entirely true…
But wait, how could I possibly love a stranger like you?

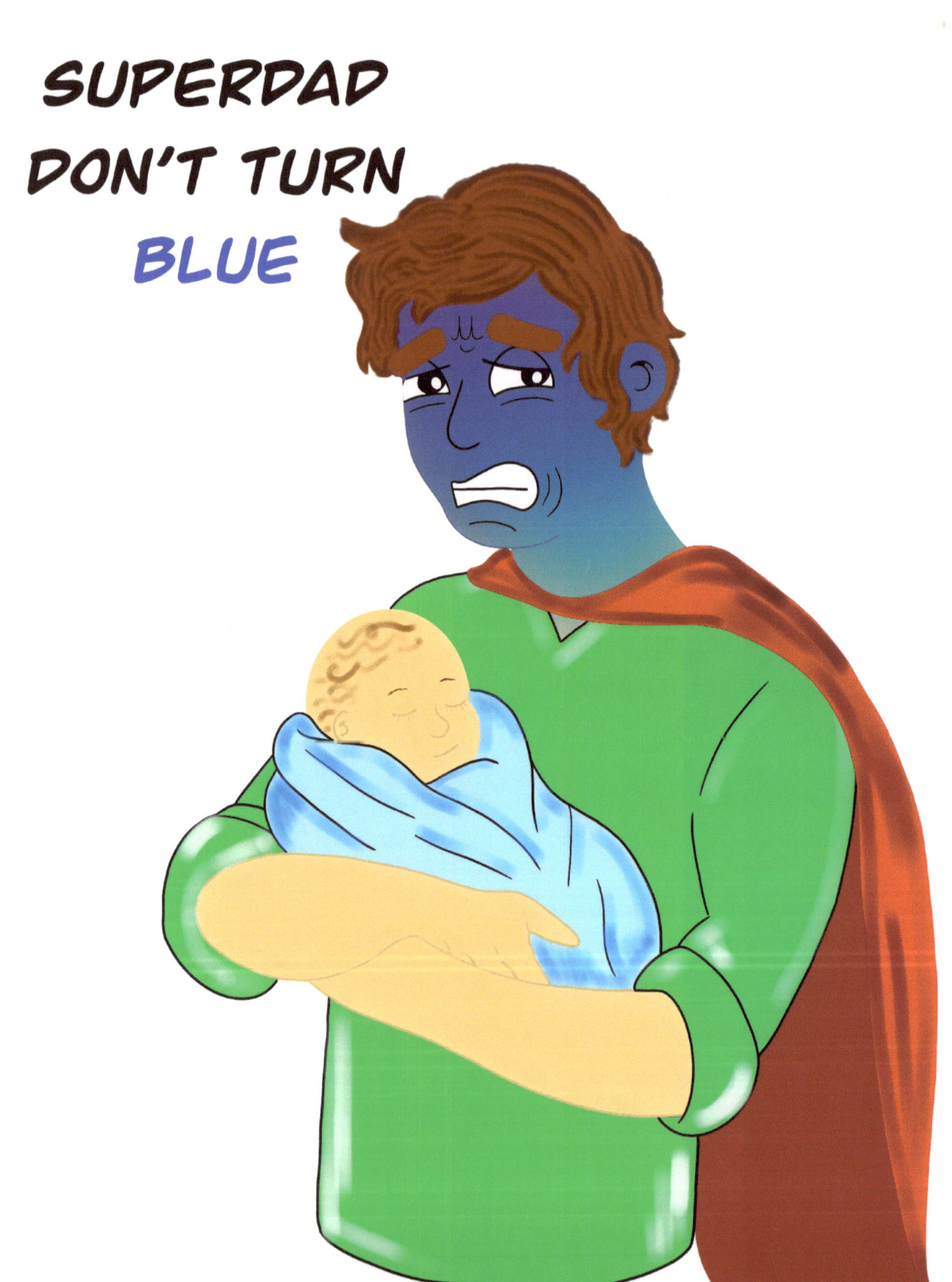

REASSURANCE

If only I could go back to that moment,

The moment when I started to feel like a mess,
I would tell myself that:

1. What I am feeling is normal and not abnormal
2. I am strong and confident
3. I am Superdad

I would tell myself that every father goes through this,
Absolutely everyone.
It doesn't mean something is wrong with you or that you are numb.

It means that the baby you are holding is brand new.

In time, you will build a beautiful relationship just between the two of you.

So please don't feel alarmed and, Superdad, don't turn blue.
Dust off your cape and stand tall, as ahead there is a lot of fun and work to do.

Remember this moment.
Cherish it well.
Trust what I am telling you as all is good and well.

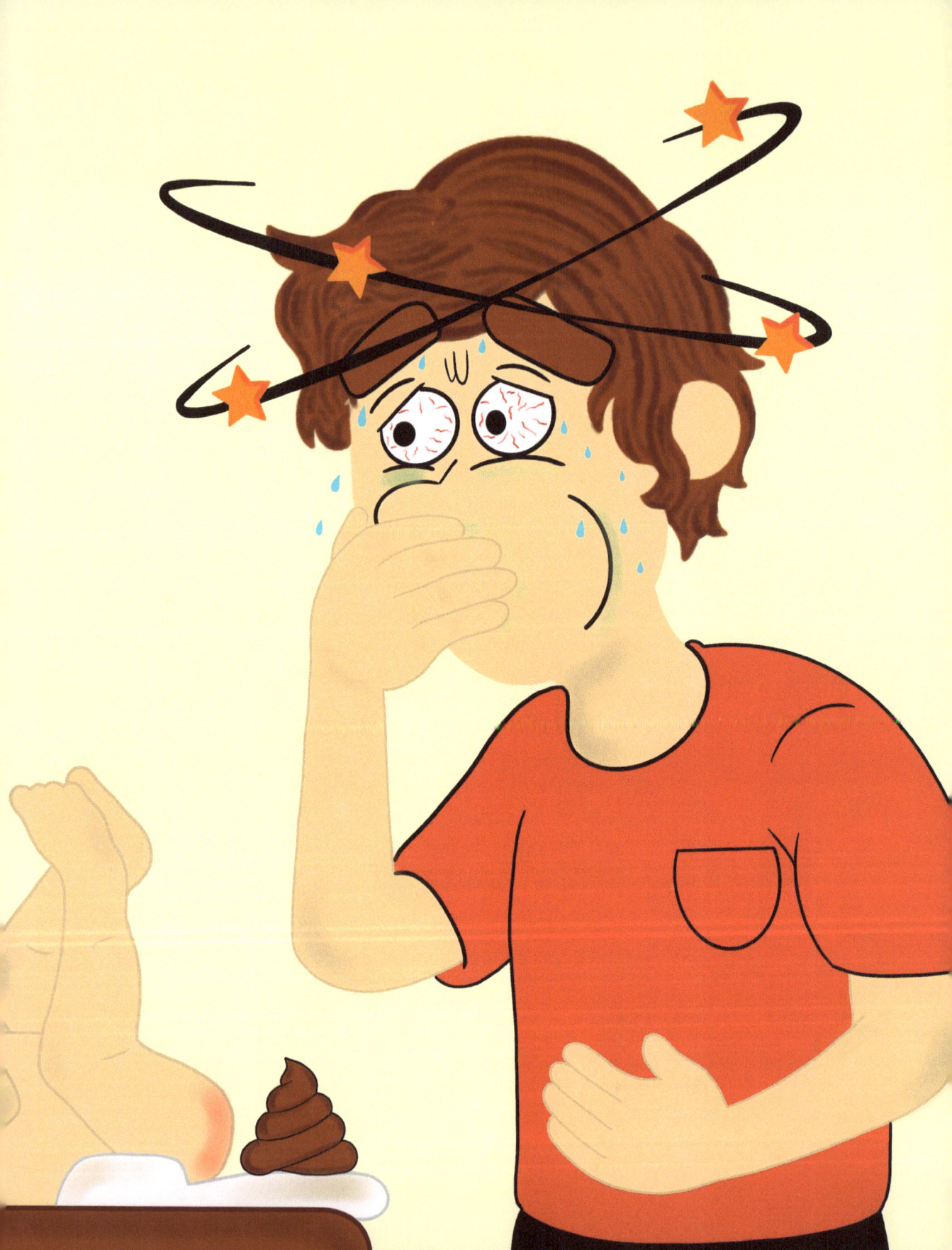

When all the visitors had gone home,
It was just you, mum and me sitting all alone.

We stared at you for what felt like hours.
It was just too surreal for us to believe we had become parents.

But now that you are here, I just don't know what to do.
I'm not even sure if I love you.
So, I tried to be the useful dad I am meant to be.
I even volunteered to change your first nappy.
I told everyone to gather around.
Watch Superdad—he will make you proud.

But with each button I'd undone,
I could not prevent what was going to come.
And when I finally opened up your nappy,
It was as if someone had sucker punched me.

Oh my God, the pong!
Where could it have possibly come from?
You, my darling, are way too small to create something so pungy...
Oh, catch me, I am about to fall!

Oh, this is madness, yes siree!
That's it, from this day on, I am never going to change another nappy.

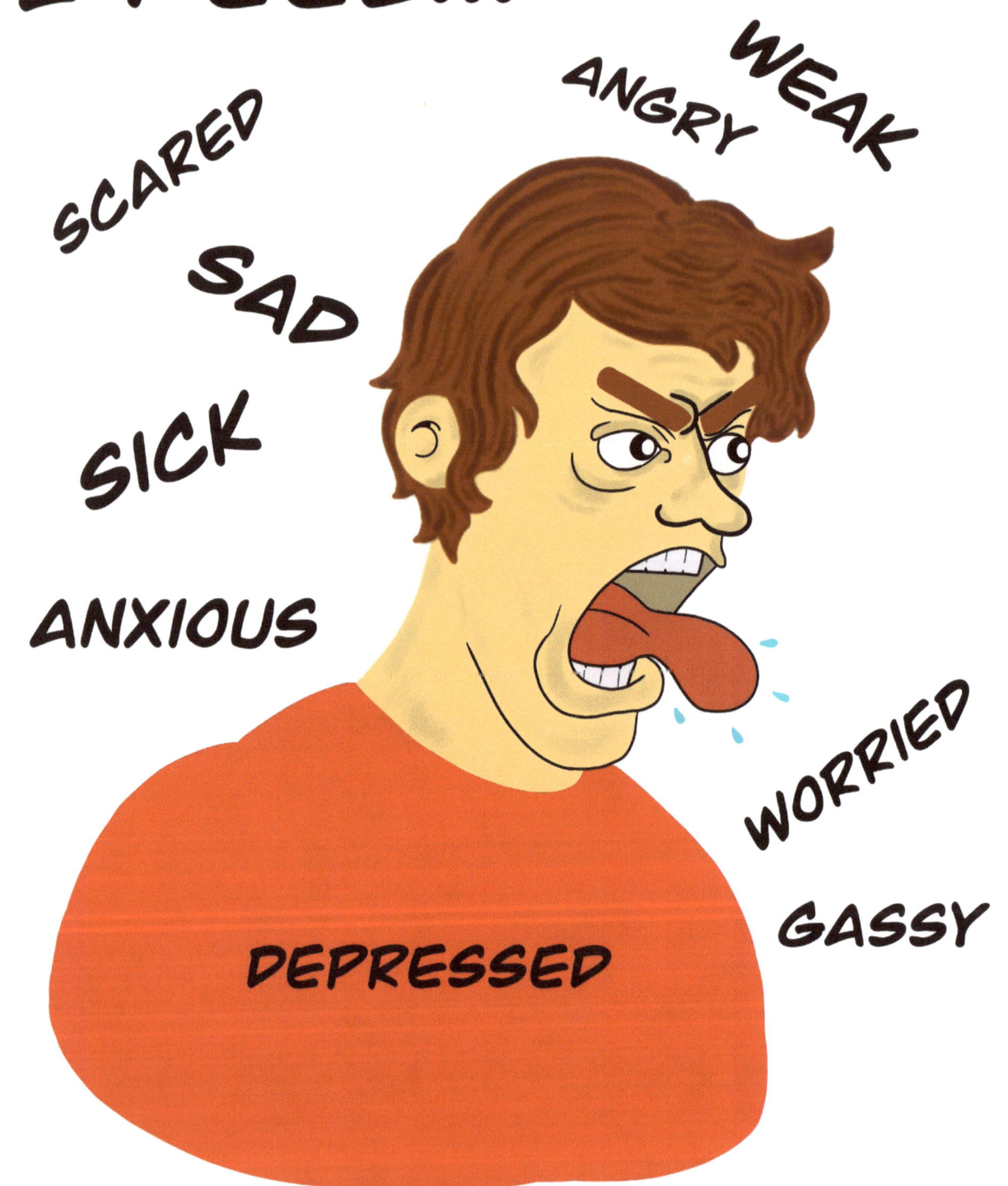

REASSURANCE

If only I could go back to that moment,
The moment when I started to feel like a mess,
I would tell myself that:

1. What I am feeling is normal and not abnormal
2. I am strong and confident
3. I am Superdad

I would tell myself to please speak up.
Shout out what you feel.
Everyone's experience is different so don't beat yourself up, you dill.

Some fathers may cry and say love at first sight.
Others may jump for joy.
And if you don't feel this, Superdad—it's okay, my boy.

So, get up.
Make sure you stand tall.
And don't forget to dust off your cape because I guarantee you,
You are going to have a ball.

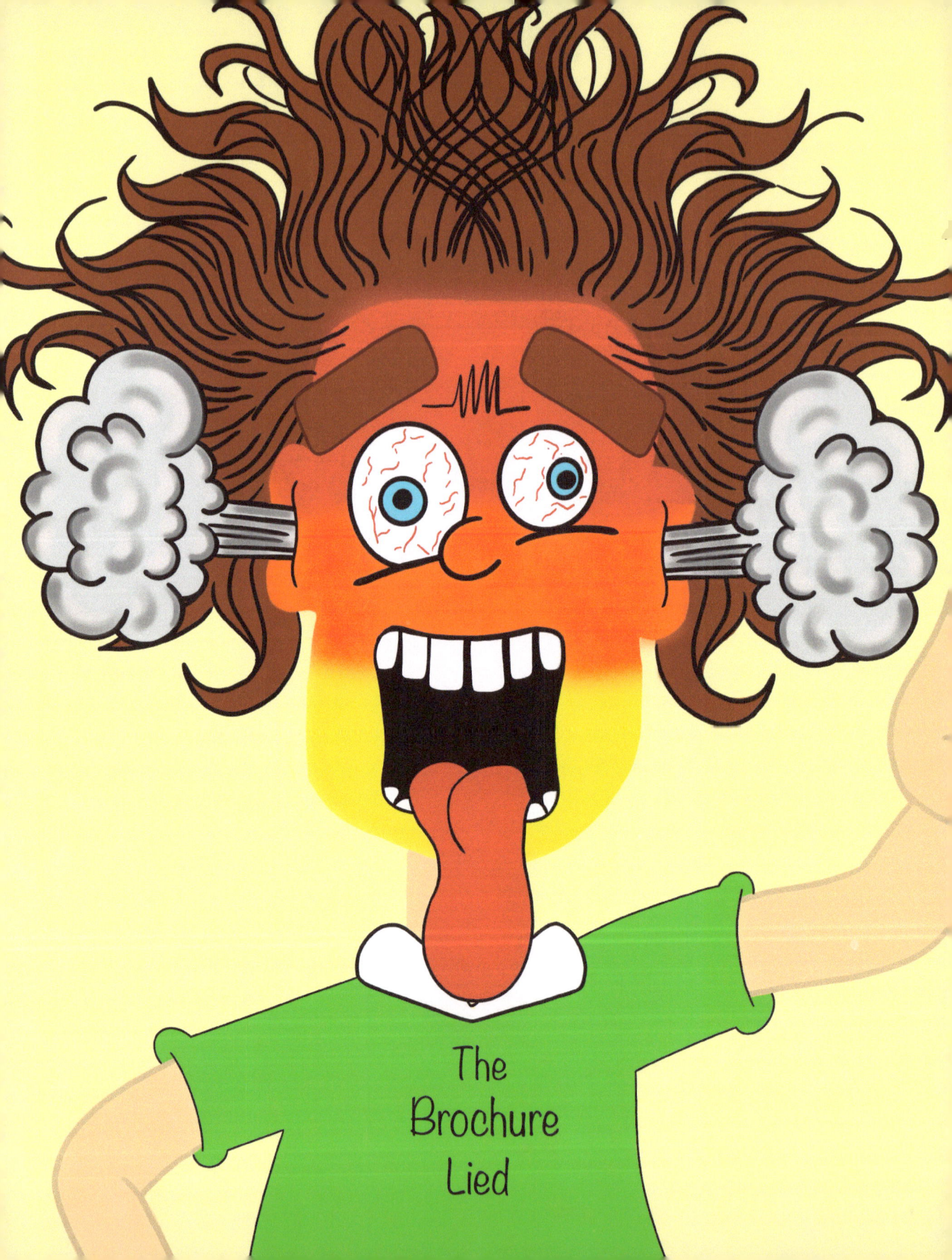

Before we knew it, it was time to go home.
It was time to leave the hospital, oh no!

I am not sure if I am ready.
There is so much doubt,
Even my stomach is churning really loud.

Oh goodness, I feel sick.
Can someone please pull the cord—call the doctor quick!

Do we have to go?
Really, do we need to leave?
Can't we stay for one more night or even one more week?

I have questions,
So many questions to ask.
And I am not sure where I am meant to start.

But our bags are packed and it's time to go.
Oh boy, I have to stand tall and take charge of this show.
I guess I need to "Man Up" then everything will be okay.

We finally arrived home.
Even though the hospital was a short drive,
Only five minutes to be precise…

I was so nervous while I steered the car.
I even had the shakes, the sweats and I needed to rip a fart.

We unloaded the car, including the baby,
Took a deep breath and entered the house ever so gladly.
But we looked at each other as we walked through the door and wondered…
What are we meant to do?
I don't know about you, but I don't have a clue.
I already have so many unanswered questions,
Questions which I desperately needed to ask.
And to top it all off, now I feel more uncertain, lost and aghast.

The first night was interesting (to say the least),
As interesting as anything new can be.
We both couldn't wait to rest and sleep ever so soundly.

But the minute we placed you in your cot,
You lit right up and said, "Sorry, mum and dad, there is no time for rest!"
In fact, there will be no sleep, as this will become our regular nightly fest.

So, you cried and cried all night long.
The strange thing is you didn't want a boob or a lullaby song.
We walked you up and down and through the house.
We took turns,
And even both had a few meltdowns.

I asked myself for the hundredth time,
"Why is my baby the one who is crying?"
No one mentioned this at all...
Is something broken?
Oh my, quick—who should we call?

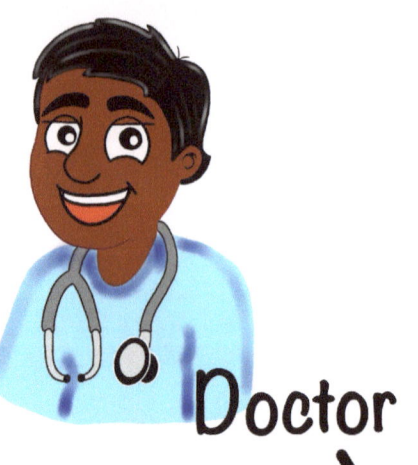
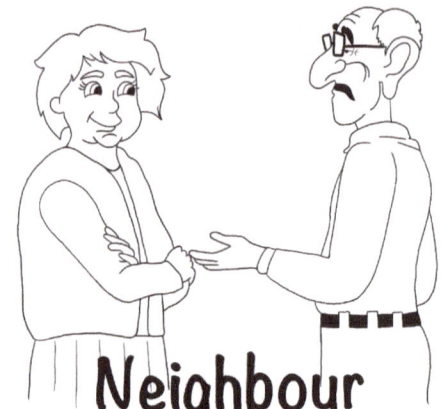

Doctor   Neighbour

Community

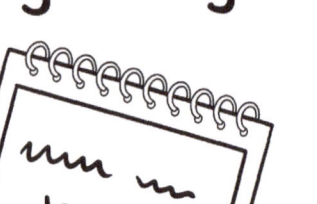
Psychologist   Nurse   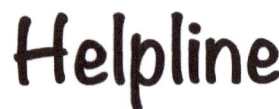 Helpline

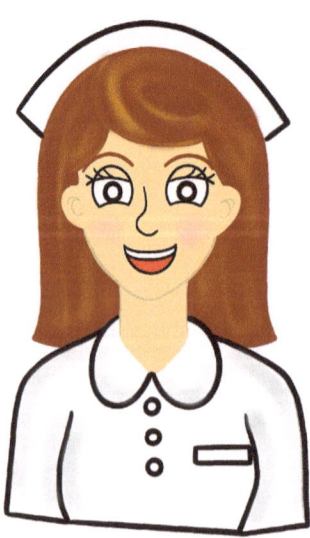
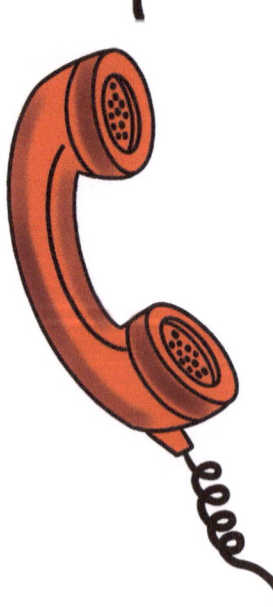

REASSURANCE

If only I could go back to that moment,
The moment when I started to feel like a mess,
I would tell myself that:

1. What I am feeling is normal and not abnormal
2. I am strong and confident
3. I am Superdad

I would tell myself to please speak up.
Tell people how you genuinely feel.
The answer isn't to "Man Up" as that isn't genuine or real.

You already are a man who is quite capable.
So, remember, Superdad, you can get up after you fall.

So, get up, Superdad, and dust off your magnificent cape.
There are plenty of people in your Community,
Whom you can reach out to any time of the day.

When the sun rose early the next day,
That's when you decided that's enough play,
As it was time for you to dream away.

But for me, there was no pillow and no bed,
No warm blanket,
And definitely no dreams to be dreamt.
Instead, it was time for me to get dressed and head off to work.

I was so exhausted.
I felt weak.
My God, parenting is hard; I should have asked my boss for one week off.
One week to recover from last night's fun.
To be honest, no one told me it was going to be this hard all night long.
Hmm, I hope Wonder Woman will cope with all this while I am gone.

ONE WEEK LATER

So, we continued in this way,
Night after night and day after day.
There was just no rest anymore nor any time of the day.

Even though we both were sleep-deprived,
I could see the changes which had arrived.
At first, they were subtle and they were small,
Like a gaping hole.
It was there even though it was hard to see.
It was something that truly distressed me.

You see, Wonder Woman, you lost that sparkle in your eyes,
Including the zest that you had for life.
And every time I came near,
You somehow magically disappeared.

I too wish I had magic,
Magic to make things bright.
But all I had was dread and fear, and no will left to stand and fight.

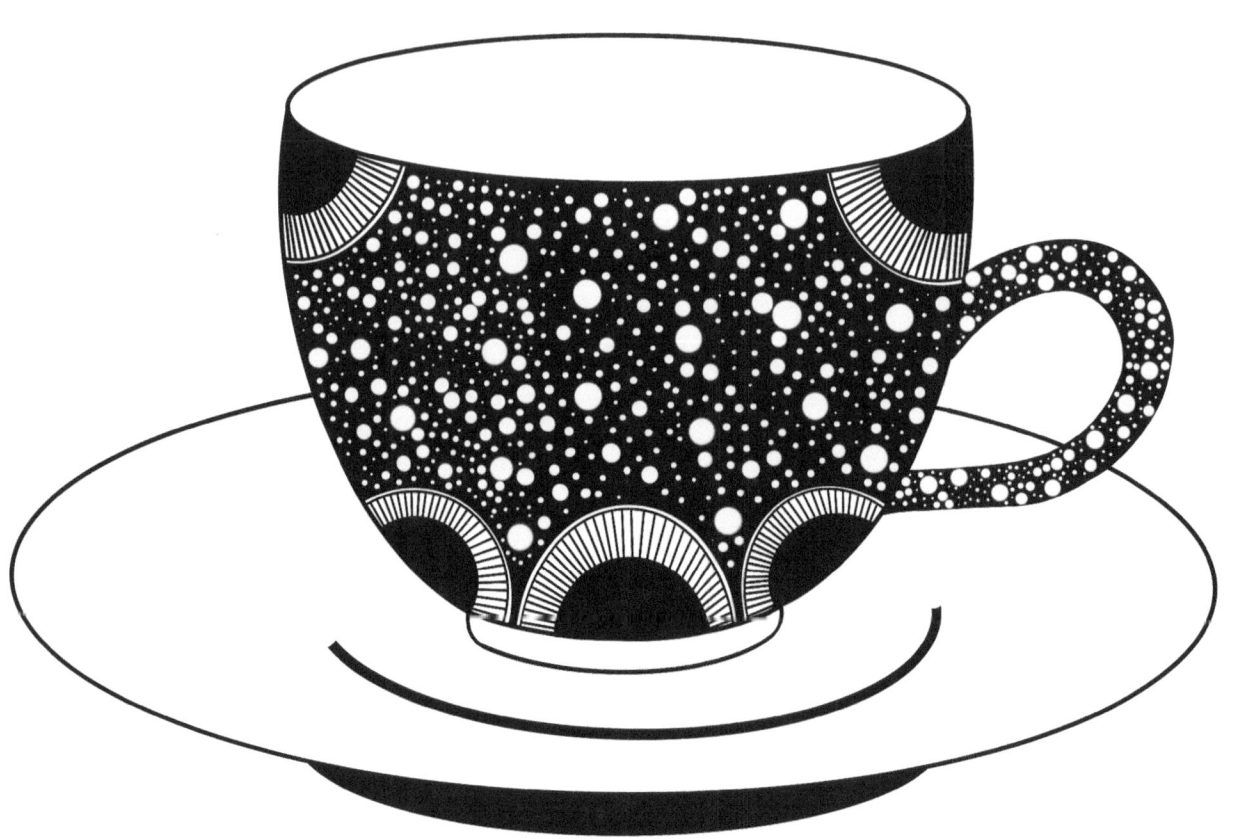

REASSURANCE

If only I could go back to that moment,
The moment when I started to feel like a mess,
I would tell myself that:

1. What I am feeling is normal and not abnormal
2. I am strong and confident
3. I am Superdad

I would tell myself to call someone and tell them what you see,
As your Wonder Woman should be sparkling not withering, dear me…

It sounds like she needs a hug and a cup of tea.
Ahh, better yet, why don't you get her to your local GP?

Sit with them and discuss how it is all going.
There is nothing wrong with saying that this is all too hard for me.

It isn't failure, oh no.
It isn't weakness, no siree.
It's simply you, Superdad, saying—can someone please help me?

Each morning, I couldn't wait to leave the house,
As I no longer could breathe.
It was just too hard to watch someone I love slowly disappear.

So, as I pulled out of the driveway,
I felt relief.
I just didn't make it very far before I heard you ring—damn, that was short-lived.

I asked myself as I started to choke, "Should I answer you?"
Perhaps today you are simply calling me to say, "I love you!"
But my belly was telling me to be aware.
So, I reluctantly answered your call and coped a berating, right then and there.
"Why aren't you here to help?"
"Why do I have to do it all by myself?"

Work was hard.
It was just so hard for me,
As I was constantly filled with an incredible amount of anxiety.

While I was there, it was hard to think.
I was constantly nervous and I felt sick.
I even felt so alone, as no one asked the father, me,
"How are you coping at home?"
Instead, everyone just placed all this pressure,
Pressure to provide.
I had to pay the bills and make sure the family survived.

But what about me?
What am I meant to show and feel?
Do I truly count or am I just meant to be strong and shut my mouth?

Am I meant to speak up?
Speak about feeling blue?
Ahh, I know, I will speak to the boys.
Surely, they will relate to what I am going through.

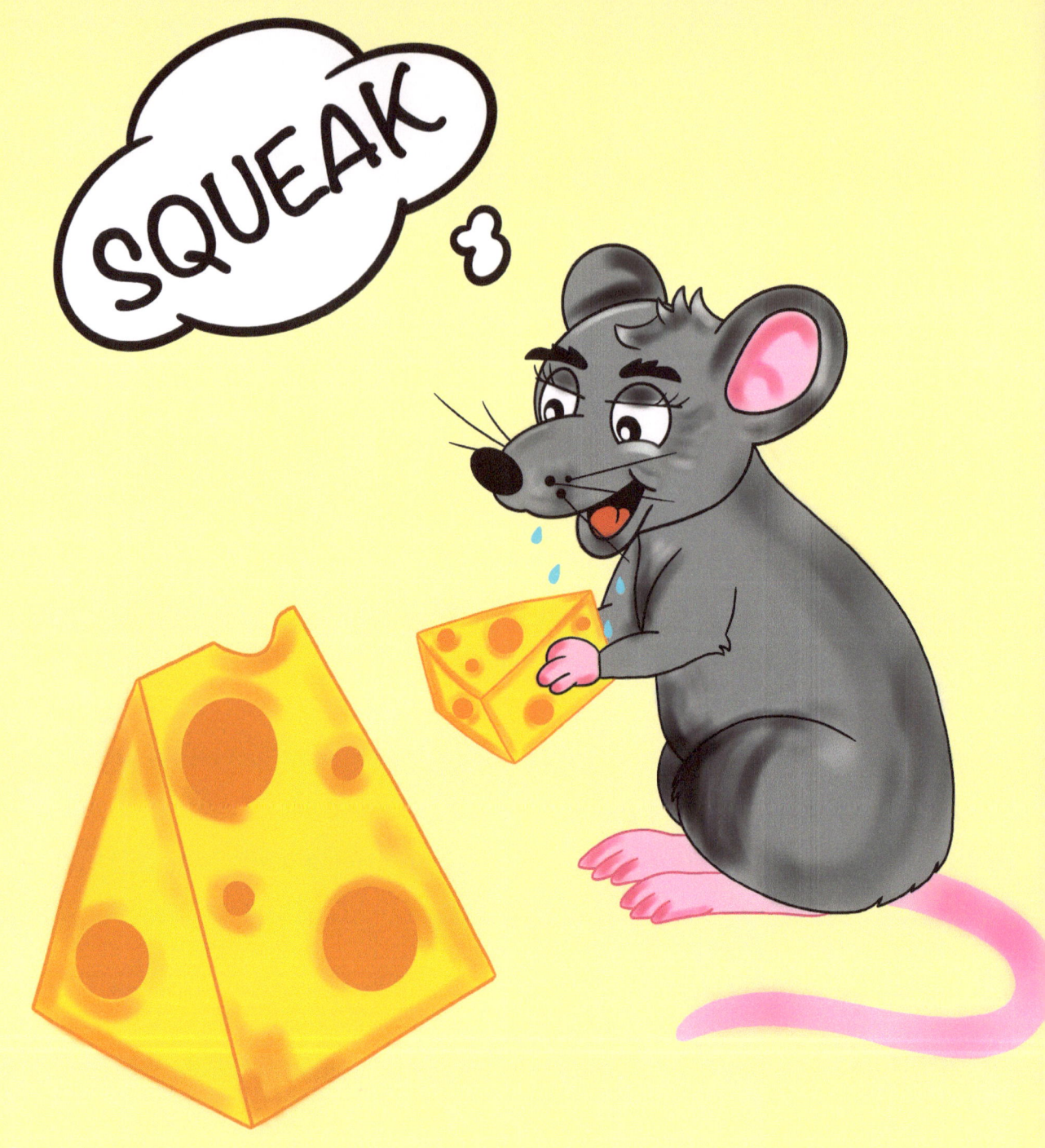

I dreaded coming home.
It was something that I desperately didn't want to do.
I stayed at work till late just to avoid the both of you.
And it wasn't because I didn't love you…

It was simply because I felt utterly crushed.
Crushed because I couldn't help you,
As it was the one thing that I, as Superdad, was clearly meant to do.
What made it worse was that I couldn't motivate you.
And it hurt my soul to say, I couldn't connect with you.

It was as if a dark cloud had descended on the house.
And instead of feeling like a Superdad,
I felt like a mouse.

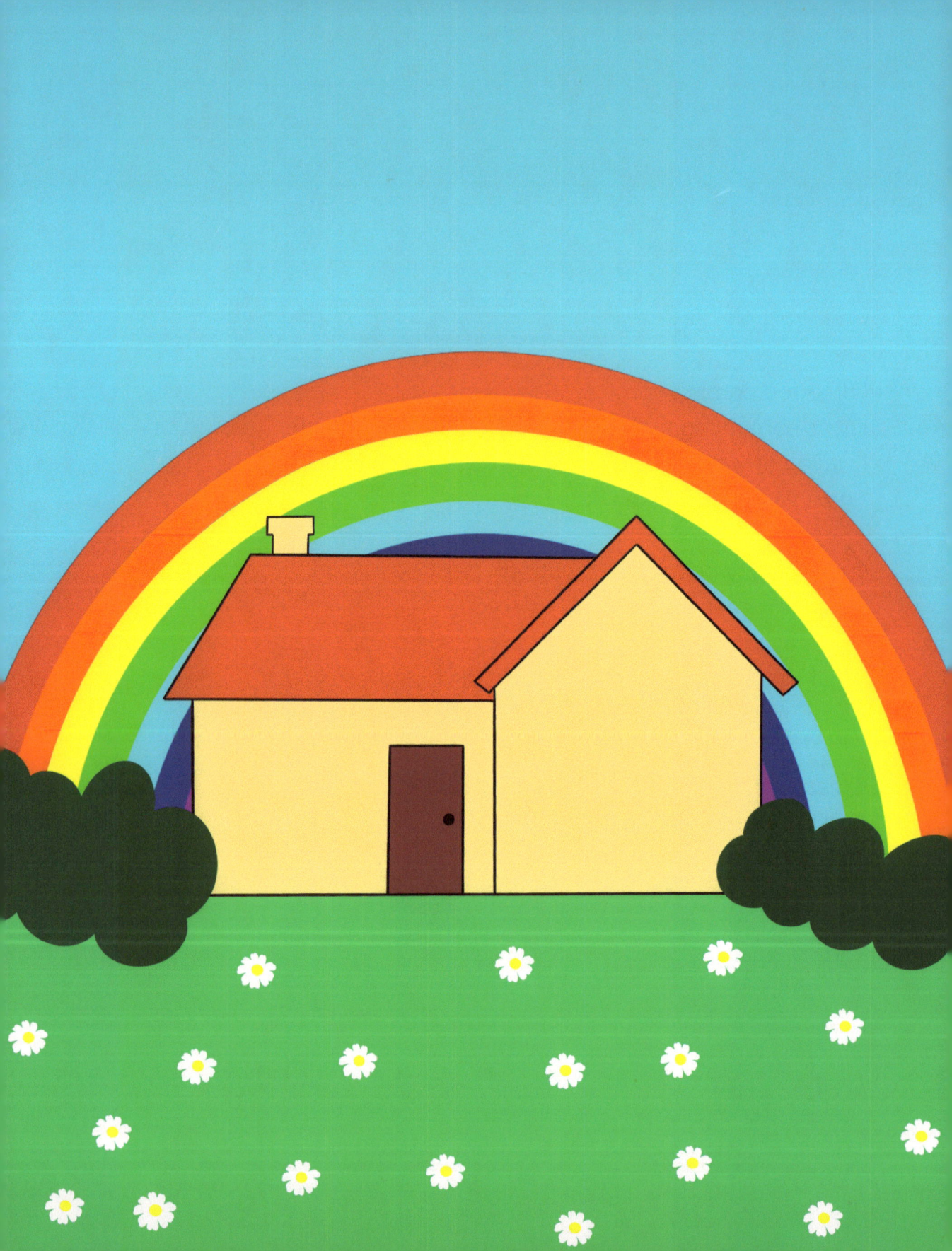

REASSURANCE

If only I could go back to that moment,
The moment when I started to feel like a mess,
I would tell myself that:

1. What I am feeling is normal and not abnormal
2. I am strong and confident
3. I am Superdad

I would tell myself that something is seriously wrong, not just with me.
You see, Wonder Woman had lost her way.
So, it's time to reach out, please…

Home should be a sanctuary,
Somewhere where you can feel at ease.
It even should be a place of love,
Not dread and unease.

Yes, sometimes we argue with the people whom we love.
But we always find a way to reconnect via a kiss and a hug.
So, if this cannot be done by absolutely anyone at home,
Please don't beat yourselves up but reach for that phone.
Then slowly, but surely, the cloud will lift from your dome.

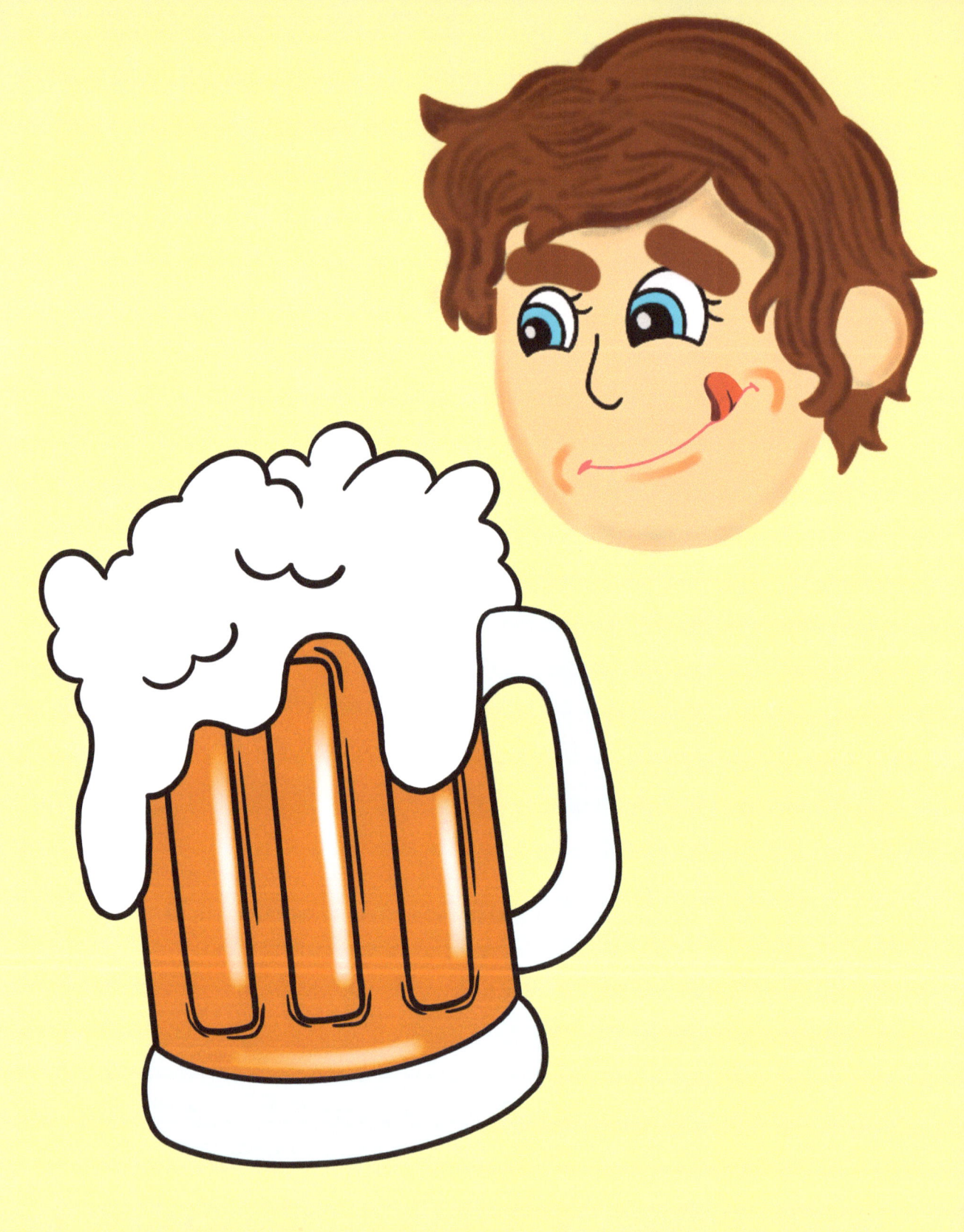

I reached for that phone.
I did dial a number,
Not to seek help but to organise a big night out.

Yes, life is tough at times but I am tougher.
All I need is a night out with the boys and some laughter.

Oh, I need a drink,
Just a small jug of beer.
I need to numb my senses and forget about the anxiety and the fear.

I need to hit the town and go to the footy.
I need to hear the roar from the crowd,
Instead of the constant cries from mum and Bub, no doubt.

I need to get away from this household,
Away from the cloud.
I need to be with my friends, where I can be normal and proud.

The night out with the boys did not go as planned,
As I didn't feel free or even proud.
All I felt was anxiety and absolute dread.
Dread from being away from home,
And away from the people who needed me more than I clearly seemed to know.

We did go to the footy but I didn't scream and shout.
To be honest, I just didn't care which team won,
Or who scored the mark of the match.
The sad thing is the beer was even a miss.
And for some reason, it lost its incredible fizz.
It felt flat in my mouth and that's when I realised I should not have gone out.

But what hurt the most, you see,
Is that the boys just didn't understand me.
I tried to talk to them about my problems.
They just brushed them off and gave me no solutions.

The next morning, I woke up feeling lifeless.
I had no desire for anything at all.
I just wanted to crawl into a deep-dark hole.

I needed someone to hold me.
Oh, please hold me tight...
Please, let this agonising feeling of hopelessness dissipate and take flight.

But as I rolled over in bed,
All I saw was my Wonder Woman looking distant, tired and crying off her head.
Oh, how can anyone at home help me and hold me tight,
When my Wonder Woman is fragile and suffering in plain sight?

I simply can't tell her how I feel.
I don't want to risk impacting on her current mental fight.
Hmm, you know what, I may be alone but I will be all right.

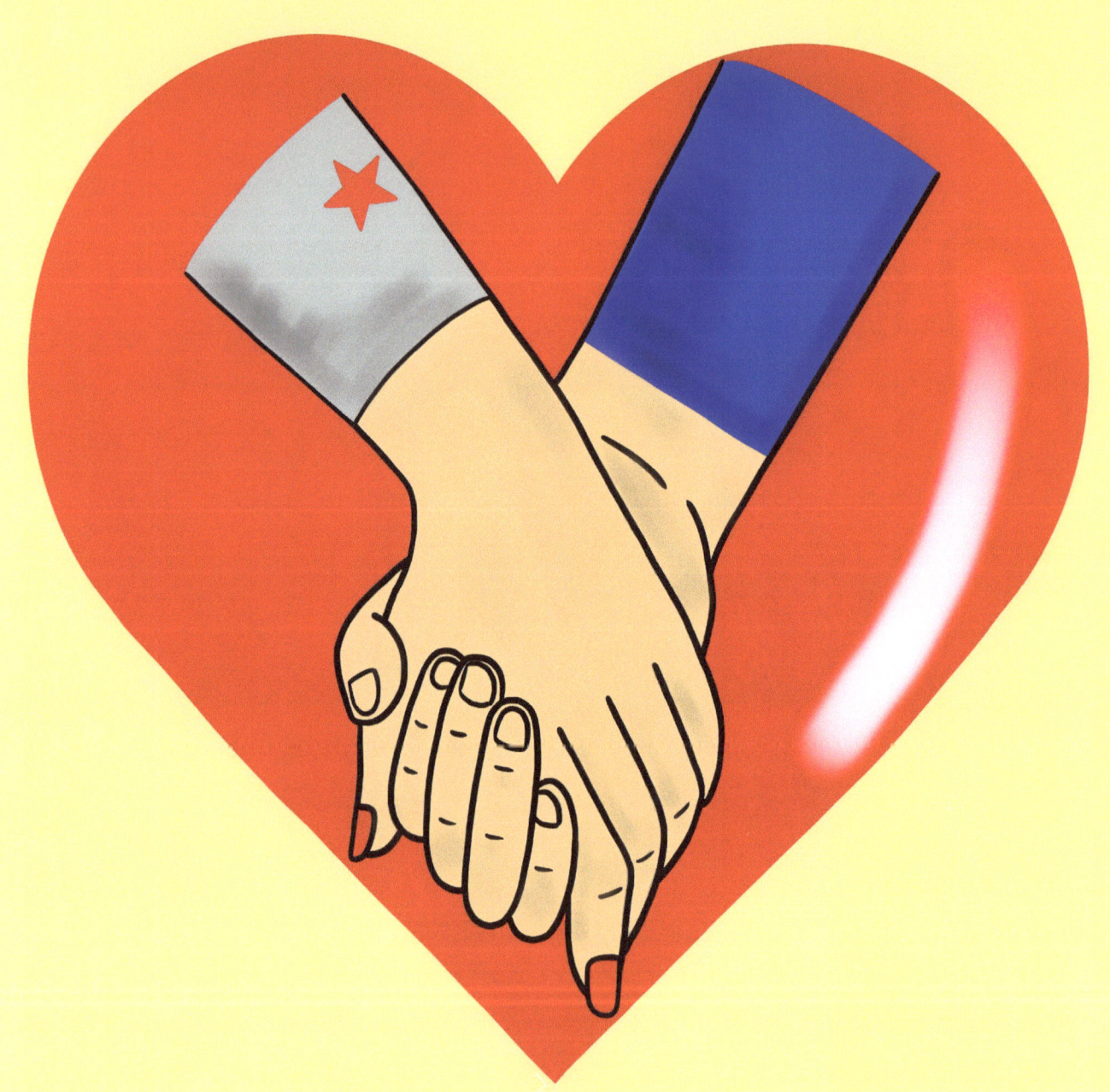

REASSURANCE

If only I could go back to that moment,
The moment when I started to feel like a mess,
I would tell myself that:

1. What I am feeling is normal and not abnormal
2. I am strong and confident
3. I am Superdad

I would tell myself that it's time.
Time which is OVERDUE!
It's time to start looking after the both of you.

You shouldn't be hurting.
You shouldn't be in pain.
You shouldn't be feeling lifeless and empty day after day.

So, get up, Superdad.
Dust off your magnificent cape.
Take your Wonder Woman by the hand,
And go grab that much needed help, as it is <u>NEVER</u> too late!

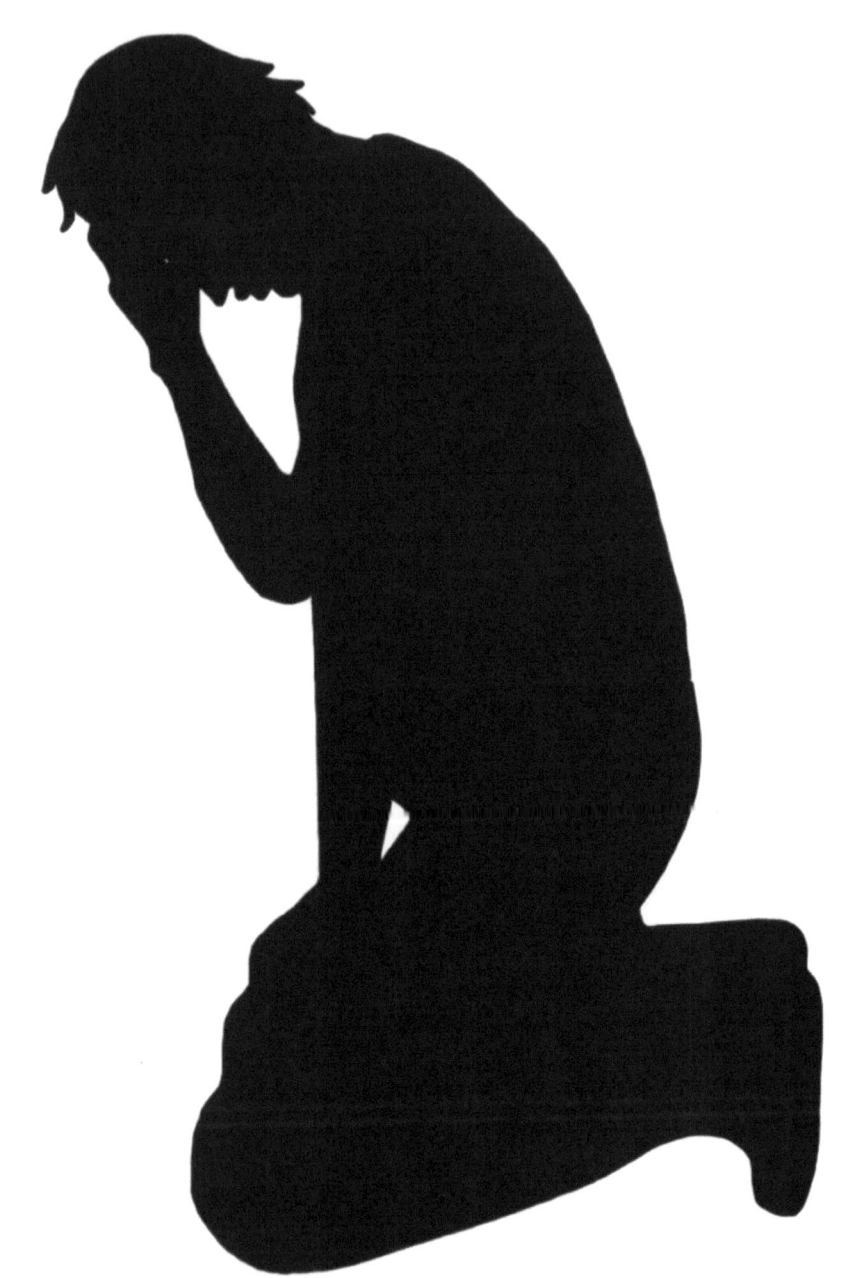

That day arrived.
It was a day of complete clarity.
It was the day I broke down and regained my dignity.

I was on my way to work,
The only place where I liked to be.
But on that day, my pain was just too much for me.

I couldn't jump out of my car.
I didn't make it to my office.
I just sat there behind the steering wheel, all numb and lifeless.

I cried.
I let the trapped tears fall.
I finally realised that Fatherhood shouldn't be this hard nor painful.

After I calmed down, and without a second thought,
I turned the ignition on and headed right back to the fort.

Today is the day I will tell my Wonder Woman about my pain.
We need to stand together.
We need to be brave.
We need to be honest,
And get help without delay.

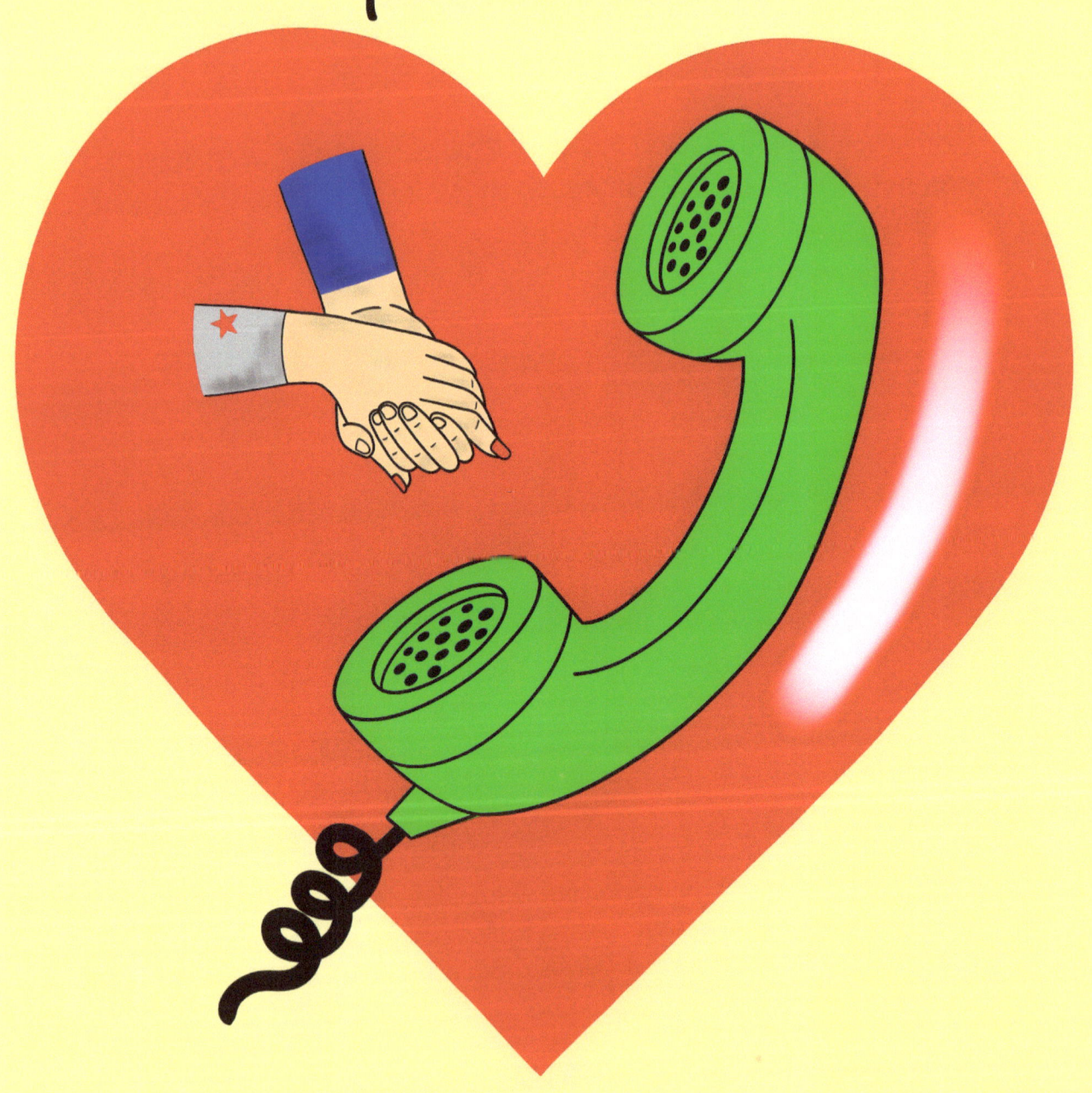

I couldn't wait to get home.
I couldn't wait to set myself free.
I couldn't wait to finally hold my darling wifey.

I raced into the driveway.
I kicked down the door.
I grabbed her by the shoulders and began to cry even more.

I held her tight and I whispered in her ear.
I told my Wonder Woman all she needed to hear.

We cried together,
Right there on the floor.
We opened up our hearts,
And broke down all our walls.

And *together* we made that phone call.

Here are their details, so just reach out...

Emergency:
000
If you or someone else is seriously injured or in need of urgent medical help, call triple zero immediately.

Gidget Foundation:
1300 851 758
www.gidgetfoundation.org.au
Supports the emotional well-being of expectant and new parents.

PANDA:
1300 726 306
www.panda.org.au
Supports families affected by anxiety and depression.

Mensline Australia:
1300 789 978
www.mensline.org.au
Provides telephone and online counselling services and offers support for Australian Men everywhere.

Beyond Blue:
1300 224 363
www.beyondblue.org.au
Provides information and support to help everyone achieve their best mental health.

Lifeline:
13 11 14
www.lifeline.org.au
Provides access to 24-hour crisis support.

What I Needed

The Biggest Needs For Husbands:

1. Drop around a meal
2. Hang out a basket of washing
3. Take the baby out for a walk
4. Be generous by washing the dishes or tidying up the house
5. Do all of the above things again the next day

The most precious gift you can give a partner (mum and dad) who is suffering is <u>Time</u>.

www.ingramcontent.com/pod-product-compliance
Lightning Source LLC
Chambersburg PA
CBHW041427010526
44107CB00045B/1529